A PR⊙-LIFE GUIDE TO BIRTH CONTROL

JUSTINA VAN MANEN

ISBN: 978-1-998170-21-0

Published and distributed by Christian Heritage Press
www.christianheritagepress.ca

Cover design by Sharon Phelps

Contents

Introduction

For Christians, the topic of birth control is one of many layers. Christians have traditionally opposed its use for several reasons.[1] In the first place, Christians focus on abstinence until marriage, protecting the virtue of both man and woman, as well as the future of any child they may conceive together. Sexual intercourse is a gift to be enjoyed only by a man and a woman within the marriage covenant. The commandment, "Thou shalt not commit adultery," is meant to keep us from damaging this gift, as well as ensure that children will be born into a loving family unit. God's commandments are good and perfect (Psalm 19: 7-10), meant to protect us from ourselves. The advent of birth control—the most recognizable form being the pill—played a key part in initiating the sexual revolution of the 1960s. When sex happens outside of marriage, the resulting children are often not seen as a gift but an unwelcome liability. Birth control allowed for a divorce between sex and pregnancy, turning sex into a purely recreational activity.

While Christian teaching is generally clear in

---

[1] The Roman Catholic Church, in particular, has made their stance on birth control very clear. Their position is explained in Pope Paul VI's *Humanae vitae* in 1968.

condemning the use of birth control outside of marriage for recreational sex, the use of birth control within marriage has been the subject of more debate over the past century. There is a wide range of views on this topic, from advocates of the "quiverfull" movement, which condemns the use of any type of family planning—including a woman tracking her cycle in what is generally known as natural family planning (NFP)—to those who see no issue with married couples purposely refraining from having any children at all. The Bible is not silent on these issues, but the range of circumstances facing couples makes it impossible to have a clear set of rules dictating what each family should look like.

The overarching guideline in family life must always be to prayerfully trust in God, giving thanks for the children that are received out of His hand, and seeking for guidance and wisdom in how to deal with each situation. Thomas Jacomb, an English Presbyterian minister who lived from 1622-1687, wrote: "Providence is not more seen in any of the affairs of men than in this of children; that there shall be many or few, some or none, all falls under the good pleasure and disposal of God." When we attempt to remove Providence from our lives and family planning, a dangerous precedent is created.

The purpose of this book is not to outline how couples ought to approach having children. Rather, it is to highlight how couples and individuals *should not* go about planning their families.

In presenting the evidence that hormonal birth control is potentially harmful to pre-born children, the intent is not to condemn those who are utilizing one of these methods or have used one in the past. The information available about birth control, either from doctors, books, or online material, is often contradictory and difficult to wade through. Those of us who are not familiar with medical terminology may struggle with how words are used and defined. This book intends to untangle these knots and provide a clear picture of what hormonal birth control is and how it works so that couples can prayerfully make decisions surrounding its use in a way that does not violate the law of God — decisions that are fundamentally pro-life.

1

What is birth control?

"I have four children ages four and under. I'm overwhelmed."
"After my previous two pregnancies, I suffered from crippling post-partum depression. I want to ensure that I am mentally healthy before I have another child."
"My husband has to travel a lot for his job. There is a limit to how many children I can handle on my own."
"I have had an aggressive form of cancer and have to be scanned every six months to ensure it hasn't returned. I'm afraid that if I get pregnant and the cancer comes back, chemotherapy could hurt or kill my baby."

***

Discussions surrounding the use of birth control are often more complex than how they are framed. People seek to prevent pregnancy for many different reasons. Some use birth control because they are unmarried, some because they don't feel ready for a child, some because they only want two children, and others because they want no children at all. There are valid reasons to avoid pregnancy and there are invalid reasons. Whatever our reason, it is important that we understand what birth control is and how it works.

Before diving into a discussion of birth control and explaining how it effectively disrupts a woman's reproductive system, it may be helpful to review how the healthy female body functions. Every month, a woman's body prepares itself to nurture the life of a new human being in what is called the menstrual cycle. The menstrual cycle consists of two main phases; the exact length of each phase varies from woman to woman. The Follicular Phase (generally days 1-14) starts with menstruation and ends with ovulation. This phase begins with the first day of a woman's period. The bright red bleeding is a result of the uterine lining being shed. While the bleeding continues, the ovaries are preparing to release an egg in a process called ovulation. The pituitary gland, located at the base of the brain, releases the hormone FSH (follicle-stimulating hormone). FSH causes follicles to rise on the surface of the ovary. One of these follicles (fluid-filled bumps) will develop a single mature egg; in the case of fraternal twins, two or more follicles produce an egg. The follicle produces the hormone estrogen, which steadily increases, peaking one to two days before ovulation.

During the second part of this first phase, once the body has completed shedding the old uterine lining, a new lining begins to develop. This lining is called the endometrium, and it becomes thicker and more enriched with blood as the time of ovulation approaches. The high levels of estrogen stimulate the production of GnRH (gonadotropin-releasing hormone), which prompts the pituitary gland to secrete LH (luteinizing hormone). The combination of LH and FSH causes the mature egg to be released from the follicle.

The Follicular Phase of the menstrual cycle ends with ovulation (days 12-14). The egg is released from the ovary and enters a woman's fallopian tubes. If sperm is present, this is where the egg may be fertilized to create an embryo. If sperm is not present, the unfertilized egg will disintegrate after approximately 24 hours. The egg-releasing follicle seals itself over and is called the corpus luteum.

The Luteal Phase takes up days 15-28 and is the final phase of the menstrual cycle. FSH and LH decrease after the release of an egg. The corpus luteum produces progesterone, which prevents the endometrial lining from being shed, creating a healthy, nutrient-rich environment for an embryo. If fertilization has occurred, the embryo will travel down the fallopian tubes into the uterus, where it may implant into the uterine wall. If fertilization does not occur, the corpus luteum disintegrates, progesterone levels drop, and the endometrial lining begins to shed, beginning the first day of a new cycle.

Stages of the Menstrual Cycle

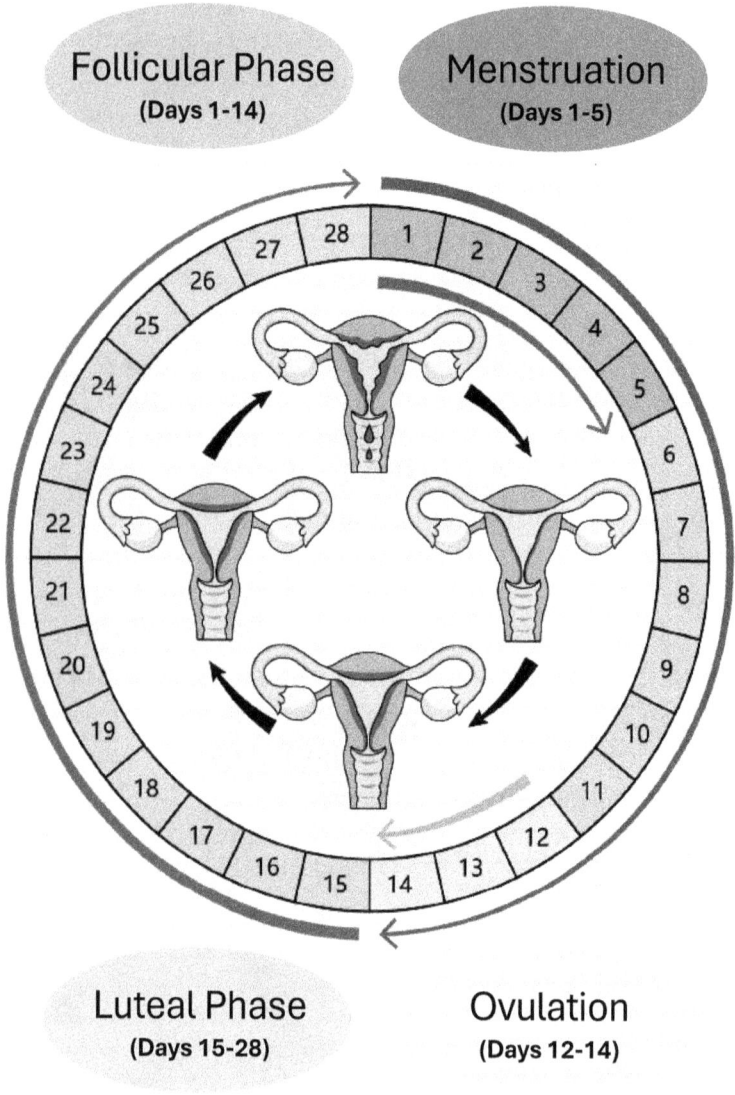

Follicular Phase
(Days 1-14)

Menstruation
(Days 1-5)

Luteal Phase
(Days 15-28)

Ovulation
(Days 12-14)

When we begin a discussion about birth control, it is essential to define our terms. In health class, at the doctor's office, and in counselling rooms, different words are used to describe how people prevent pregnancy. When birth control is mentioned, it is an overarching term, defined by *Merriam-Webster Dictionary* as follows:

birth control
1. control of the number of children or offspring born especially by preventing or lessening the frequency of conception: CONTRACEPTION
2. contraceptive devices or preparations

Using the first definition, birth control includes Plan B (also known as the morning-after pill), RU-486 (also known as the abortion pill), and abortion.[2] However, most people refer to birth control in the context of the second definition—contraception. The dictionary defines contraception as the deliberate prevention of conception or impregnation.

When differentiating between contraception and birth control, most understand the difference as follows: "[a]ll types of contraception are forms of birth control, but contraceptive forms are more spe-

---

[2] MedicalDictionary.com, Accessed Sept 2022, refers to these methods as methods of contragestion, that is: "Any contraceptive method that specifically prevents the gestation of a fertilized egg... either by making the implantation site uninhabitable or by promoting the fertilized product's expulsion."

cific in that they are used for the purpose of preventing sperm from reaching a female's egg."[3] The most logical way to break down this word would be to call it *contraception*. While this may be the general understanding of these terms, it is essential to note that the definition includes both conception *and* impregnation.

Conception is defined as:

> the process of becoming pregnant involving **fertilization or implantation or both** (emphasis added)

Impregnation is defined as:

> to make pregnant: FERTILIZE

By including both the words fertilization and implantation, the word conception can mean two very different things. When fertilization and conception are used interchangeably, they refer to the process where a sperm penetrates an egg, creating a whole, distinct, living individual. However, when conception is used interchangeably with implantation, it refers to an event that generally takes place 8-9 days *after* fertilization. During this period, the

---

[3] Corlis, Nick. "Difference Between Protection, Birth Control, & Contraception," *Exposed,* stdcheck.com, September 16, 2015, https://www.stdcheck.com/blog/difference-between-protection-birth-control-and-contraception/

newly created embryo travels down a woman's fallopian tubes and implants in the uterine wall. While the literal definition of impregnation indicates that a woman is pregnant at the moment of fertilization, many do not consider a woman "impregnated" until after the embryo has attached himself/herself to the uterine wall.[4]

Going through these definitions, it is difficult to decide whether they add clarity or confusion, and it is natural to ask: Does it matter which words we use? Yes, it matters. It is not an overstatement to say that the lives of tiny, vulnerable children depend on how we understand this terminology. For Christians who believe that life must be protected from its very beginning to its natural end, it is essential to understand when life begins, and how doctors and others understand this beginning. When a doctor or nurse practitioner states that a form of birth control does not end a pregnancy, do they believe a woman is pregnant at fertilization or not until implantation? If they are referring to implantation— which is true in many cases—they are not acknowledging that a tiny human being came into existence 8-9 days prior to this event.

The choice to use the word birth control rather than contraception is intentional because, while contraception can refer to the prevention of implantation, if it is used in the way that was originally intended (*contra-conception*) and in the way it is still

---

[4] Pregnancy cannot be medically detected until after implantation and HCG (the pregnancy hormone) can be traced with early blood tests.

often understood, it describes "barrier methods" such as male and female condoms, diaphragms, cervical caps, and spermicide gels, as well as more permanent measures such as tubal ligation ("tubes tied") and vasectomies.

While using a barrier method—which focuses on ensuring that the sperm never reaches the egg so that fertilization never occurs—has moral implications for couples both inside and outside of marriage, these types of contraception are not problematic in the same way that hormonal birth control methods are. Barrier methods do not endanger or potentially end the lives of innocent human beings, making their use a moral issue rather than a justice issue. On the other hand, while hormonal methods of birth control such as the implant, IUD, shot, vaginal ring, patch, and the pill have the primary purpose of preventing fertilization from occurring, they also have mechanisms of action that ensure that if fertilization does happen the embryo is unable to thrive in his/her mother's uterus. This reality makes the use of hormonal birth control not only a moral issue but also a justice issue because the lives of innocent human beings are at stake.

The fact that hormonal birth control does not only *prevent* pregnancy but can also *end* pregnancy is not something that is commonly understood. Many healthcare professionals will deny that this is the case, and the confusion of terms is most often the cause of this misunderstanding. Many doctors, nurses, and medical journals refer not to embryos but to "fertilized eggs," "fertilized products," or "the conceptus." Dr. Maureen Condic, an American neurobiology professor, bioethicist, and appointee to the United States' National Science Board, wrote in her paper "When Does Human Life Begin?" that in reality, there is no such thing as a "fertilized egg." Condic explains that at the moment of fertilization, the sperm and egg cells no longer exist, and a cell genetically distinct from both parent cells is created. Condic wrote:

> Based on [the] factual description of the events following sperm-egg binding, we can confidently conclude that a new cell, the zygote, comes into existence at the "moment" of sperm-egg fusion, an event that occurs in less than a second. At the point of fusion, sperm and egg are physically united – i.e., they cease to exist as gametes, and they form a new entity that is materially distinct from either sperm or egg. The behavior of this new cell also differs radically from that of either sperm or egg: the developmental pathway entered into by the zygote is distinct from both gametes. Thus, sperm-egg fusion is indeed a scientifically well defined "instant" in which the zygote... is formed.[5]

As Randy Alcorn wrote in his book *Does the Birth Control Pill Cause Abortions?*, "As the sperm no longer exists, neither in essence does the egg. It is

---

[5] Condic, Maureen. "When Does Human Life Begin?" *The Westchester Institute For Ethics & the Human Person, White Paper Volume 1, Number 1* (October 2008). pg. 5.

replaced by a new creation with unique DNA, rapidly growing and dividing on its own. This new human being is no more a mere 'fertilized egg' than it is a 'modified sperm.'"[6] The words we use matter. When a doctor tells a woman that the birth control she uses both "prevents fertilization and promotes the expulsion of the products of fertilization," few would understand this to mean the initiation of an early miscarriage. That is, however, precisely what it does mean.

The waters have been purposefully muddied in an effort to conceal the cost pre-born children pay for men and women to have "control" over their sexuality and family plans. This makes clarifying terms essential. Life begins at fertilization, the moment of sperm-egg fusion. What is created in this moment is not a fertilized egg but an embryo. An embryo is a whole, distinct, living human being, created in the image of God. If hormonal birth control fails to prevent fertilization, and the conceived child is subsequently unable to implant in the thinned uterine lining, the child, intentionally or unintentionally, becomes a very early or young victim of abortion.

---

[6] Alcorn, Randy. *Does the Birth Control Pill Cause Abortions?* 11th edition (2011), pg. 15.

2

How does it work?

"We need to discuss birth control," Sarah's doctor told her. "Have you taken anything before?"

"I took the pill for a couple months when I was a teenager to regulate my period," Sarah replied. "But I'd rather not take it again."

"How about an IUD? Of course, I'm assuming you don't want to get pregnant again in the near future."

"Well, no, at least not until our youngest is older. But I'm not sure I'm comfortable with an IUD. Are they safe?"

"Very safe. As with everything, there can be side effects but these are generally very minor. What exactly are you worried about?"

"I've heard that birth control can cause a miscarriage. Is that true?"

The doctor smiled. "Absolutely not. Birth control prevents pregnancy – it doesn't end it. You can't have a miscarriage if you don't get pregnant in the first place, can you?"

***

For those of us who do not have a medical background, relying on medical professionals to explain how different procedures and medications work makes sense. In the case of birth control, however, we need to be careful. Conversations like this one are common. When women express their concerns, doctors often dismiss them, not necessarily because they are deliberately deceptive, but because they may have a different definition of what constitutes pregnancy. As explained in Chapter 1, the terms used are often interchangeable, making it difficult to know what exactly is meant: the prevention of fertilization or the prevention of implantation. Because of this confusion, we need to understand how the standard methods of birth control work.

Planned Parenthood, the go-to organization in the United States for information about birth control, includes in its list of methods: condoms, diaphragms, birth control sponges, spermicides and gels, cervical caps, fertility awareness, the withdrawal method, breastfeeding, outercourse, abstinence, sterilization, and vasectomies. While there are meaningful conversations that need to happen about the use of these forms of birth control, they are not the focus of this book.[7] Planned Parenthood also mentions: the birth control implant, shot, vaginal ring, patch, pill, and IUD. It is these forms of hormonal birth control that we need to highlight. How do they function?

---

[7] These types of contraception prevent sperm and egg from coming together. If they fail, they will have no negative effect on the newly-created embryo.

Birth Control Implant

The birth control implant, otherwise known as Nexplanon (there is an older version called Implanon), is a thin plastic tube similar in size to a matchstick. After it is inserted under the skin of the arm by a doctor or nurse, the implant begins to release the hormone progestin. Progestin thickens the cervical mucus, which prevents the sperm from passing through the cervix and up to the fallopian tubes. It can also prevent ovulation.[8] If an egg is not released during a woman's cycle, fertilization cannot occur. Nexplanon also changes the lining of the uterus.[9,10] One of the main selling points of the implant is its longevity: it can be effective for up to five years, though it is recommended to replace it after three.[11]

---

[8] "Birth Control Implant," *Planned Parenthood,* accessed September 2022, https://www.plannedparenthood.org/learn/birth-control/birth-control-implant-nexplanon

[9] "What is Nexplanon," *Nexplanon (etonogestrel implant) 68 mg Radiopaque,* accessed September 14, 2022, https://www.nexplanon.com/what-is-nexplanon/

[10] Mayo Clinic Staff, "Contraceptive implant," *Mayo Clinic,* June 15, 2021, https://www.mayoclinic.org/tests-procedures/contraceptive-implant/about/pac-20393619

[11] Kaunitz, Andrew, M.D., "Patient education: Hormonal Methods of birth control (Beyond the Basics)," *UpToDate,* January 29, 2021, https://www.uptodate.com/contents/hormonal-methods-of-birth-control-beyond-the-basics?csi=d35481f8-1f1b-46cc-96e4-1ebc709c811b&source=contentShare

Birth Control Shot

The birth control shot is an injection given by a health care provider in the upper arm or buttock every 12-13 weeks (3 months). Depo-Provera is the only injectable form of birth control available at this point. The shot releases progestin, thickening the cervical mucus and discouraging ovulation. It also thins the uterine lining to the point where some women receiving the shot do not have their period for several months.

Vaginal Ring

A vaginal ring is a flexible plastic ring containing both estrogen and progestin. There are two types of rings, one which needs to be replaced monthly, and one which lasts for up to a year. Monthly rings (the NuvaRing or EluRyng) are placed inside the vagina, where the hormones released are absorbed into the vaginal lining. It can be used to skip a period. The Annovera ring lasts for one year. It is placed in the vagina for 21 days (3 weeks) and then taken out for 7 days. Vaginal rings function similarly to the implant and the shot, as they prevent the ovaries from releasing an egg, thicken the cervical mucus to make it more difficult for sperm to reach the egg, and thin the uterine lining.

Birth Control Patch

Birth Control patches (such as Xulane or Twirla) contain both estrogen and progestin. The patch is worn on the skin of the upper torso, buttocks, upper outer arm, or abdomen, preventing ovulation, thickening the cervical mucus, and thinning the uterine lining. A new patch is applied once a week for three weeks and left off for the fourth week.

The Birth Control Pill

There are several different types of birth control pills (oral contraceptives). Combination pills — the most common pill — contain both estrogen and progestin. The pills are small tablets that must be taken once a day, preferably at the same time. A pack can contain 21 pills or 28 pills. In the larger packs, seven of the pills are placebo pills containing no hormones (also known as sugar pills), serving the purpose of continuing a daily habit. The pill prevents ovulation, thickens the cervical mucus, and thins the lining of the uterus.

Seasonale functions in the same way as the combination pill in that it is taken as a tablet and contains estrogen and progestin. However, rather than taking 21 active pills and seven placebo pills (or no pills at all), these packs contain 84 active pills and seven placebo pills. This means that a woman will only have a period every three months.

The mini was created for people who cannot or should not take estrogen, and only contains progestin. These pills come in 28-day packs. In one type of mini-pill (containing norethindrone), all 28 pills contain progestin. In the second type (containing drospirenone), 24 pills are active, and four pills are placebo pills. The mini-pill thickens the cervical mucus and thins the uterine lining. It may also discourage ovulation, but it is not as effective as the combination pill in doing so.

IUD

IUD stands for intrauterine device, also known as intrauterine contraception (IUC) or hormonal intrauterine system (IUS). There are two types of IUDs: hormonal and copper. There are four brands of hormonal IUDs: Mirena, Kyleena, Liletta, and Skyla. The IUD is a small piece of flexible plastic shaped like a T, containing only progestin. The Mirena and Liletta IUDs can stay in place for six to seven years; Kyleena lasts for five years, and Skyla for up to three years. In slowly releasing progestin, IUDs thicken the cervical mucus, thin the lining of the uterus, and change the endometrial chemistry, impairing a sperm's movement and function and decreasing its ability to fertilize an egg. In some people, the IUD also prevents ovulation.

The copper IUD (ParaGard) is advertised as a non-hormonal form of birth control. It is shaped in the same way as the hormonal IUDs, but is wrapped in copper wire and does not contain progestin or estrogen. The copper produces an inflammatory reaction by releasing copper ions into the uterine cavity. These ions are toxic to sperm (and potentially to embryos). They change the endometrial chemistry, making it difficult for sperm to fertilize an egg and making the uterus a hostile environment for any foreign cells. They also thicken the cervical mucus.

To summarize, methods of hormonal birth control usually function in three ways:

Hormonal birth control discourages ovulation: if no egg is released during a woman's cycle, pregnancy cannot occur (implant, shot, ring, patch, combination pill, and in some cases, IUD).

Hormonal birth control thickens the cervical mucus, making it difficult for sperm to travel to the fallopian tubes, preventing fertilization (implant, shot, ring, patch, pill, IUD).

Hormonal birth control reduces the normal monthly growth of the lining of the uterus. This ensures that if the first two functions fail, the embryo will be unable to implant in the uterine wall (implant, shot, ring, patch, pill, IUD).

Some research outlines a fourth function of birth control that is more difficult to prove but still worth mentioning. There is some evidence that hormonal birth control can affect the motility of the fallopian tubes—how the fallopian tubes contract in order to push the egg toward the uterus. In his research, Randy Alcorn discovered that "Estrogen and progestin may also alter the pattern of muscle contractions in the tubes and uterus. This may interfere with implantation by speeding up the fertilized egg's travel time so that it reaches the uterus before it is mature enough to implant." [12] John Wilks of Pharmacists for Life International wrote that the pill "causes changes to the movement of the

---

[12] Alcorn, Randy. *Does the Birth Control Pill Cause Abortions?* 11th edition (2011), pg. 64.

fallopian tubes," [13] which functions primarily to prevent fertilization from occurring. Another study found that progesterone and levonorgestrel did affect the muscular contractions in the fallopian tubes.[14]

Finally, there is evidence that if contraception fails, there is a slightly higher risk of ectopic pregnancy, where an embryo implants outside of the uterus, most commonly in the fallopian tubes.[15,16] This risk is significantly higher for those using an IUD than those taking another form of hormonal birth control.[17] An ectopic pregnancy is very dangerous for the mother, as a ruptured fallopian tube can cause severe internal bleeding, and is always fatal for the child, as the child is unable to survive outside of the uterus.

---

[13] John Wilks, "The Pill — How it Works and Fails," Pharmacists for Life Internation, Oct. 1998, https://www.pfli.org/faq_oc.html

[14] K. Wanggren et al., "Regulation of muscular contractions in the human Fallopian tubes through prostaglandins and progestagens," Oxford Academic, human reproduction, October 2008, https://academic.oup.com/humrep/article/23/10/2359/713379

[15] Cheng Li, et al., "Effects of Levonorgestrel and progesterone on Oviductal physiology in mammals," National Library of Medicine, 2018, https://www.ncbi.nlm.nih.gov/pmc/articles/PMC6011509

[16] Cheng Li, et al., "Contraceptive Use and the Risk of Ectopic Pregnancy: A Multi-Center Case-Control Study," National Library of Medicine, 2014, https://www.ncbi.nlm.nih.gov/pmc/articles/PMC4262460

[17] Yun XQ, "Relationship between ectopic pregnancy and IUD," National Library of Medicine, May 1991, https://pubmed.ncbi.nlm.nih.gov/12317373

It is worth noting that the majority of the information in this chapter came from the Planned Parenthood website (primarily based in the United States), the SHORE Centre website (the Canadian branch of Planned Parenthood), Action Canada for Sexual Health and Rights, UpToDate (a website used by many American and Canadian doctors), and the websites produced by those who created the drugs themselves. None of these websites are pro-life; in fact, most actively promote abortion. The way these forms of birth control function is not a pro-choice secret. This information is easily accessible to anyone who is looking for it—extensive drug monographs are available for free on websites such as rxlist.com, drugs.com, and Medscape. Similar to barrier methods, the first two functions of HBC listed have moral implications but not justice implications—they focus on pre-venting pregnancy rather than ending pregnancy. For the purposes of this book, it is the third function, the altering of the uterine lining (and potentially the fourth function of disrupted tubal motility) that is definitely ethically problematic.

	Prevents the ovary from releasing an egg.	Thickens cervical mucus to make it more difficult for a sperm to reach an egg.	Thins the lining of the uterus to make the implantation of an embryo more difficult.	Changes endometrial chemistry to create an inhospitable environment.
Birth Control Implant	✓	✓	✓	✗
Birth Control Shot	✓	✓	✓	✗
Vaginal Ring	✓	✓	✓	✗
Birth Control Patch	✓	✓	✓	✗
Birth Control Pill	✓	✓	✓	✗
Seasonale (Pill)	✓	✓	✓	✗
Birth Control Mini-Pill	**Sometimes**	✓	✓	✗
Hormonal IUD	**Sometimes**	✓	✓	✓
Copper IUD	✗	✓	✗	✓

3

What Birth Control can do to your Baby

"I've recently gotten an IUD," Rachel casually mentioned to her friend. "I don't want to get pregnant again until the twins are at least three or four, and my doctor recommended it as super effective. Apparently it will last for years!"
Jamie shifted uncomfortably. "Uh... didn't your doctor mention that the IUD can cause a miscarriage?"
"Oh, I asked her about that. She said it isn't true."
"Have you had lighter periods lately?"
"Yes, it's been amazing! I did have some cramping and stuff, but that's all gone now."
"Okay, did the doctor say why you might have lighter periods?"
"No, she just said it was one of the benefits of getting an IUD."
"IUDs thin the lining of your uterus; that's why most people have a lighter flow. But one of the consequences of thinning the lining is that if fertilization does happen, the embryo isn't able to implant."
"Okay, so what are you saying?"
"We know that life begins at fertilization, right?"
"Yes..."

> *"Well, if the IUD doesn't manage to prevent*
> *ovulation or the sperm from reaching the egg,*
> *fertilization can still happen. The baby just can't*
> *implant in the uterine wall. That means it's possible*
> *your IUD could cause an early miscarriage."*
> *Rachel looked shocked, then angry. "Why didn't my*
> *doctor tell me that? She knows I'm pro-life and would*
> *never want to hurt my baby!"*

***

Hormonal forms of birth control — without exception — thin the endometrial lining. Many resources list this as one of the benefits of being on birth control. While it may be convenient or, due to certain health conditions, beneficial for a woman taking birth control to have a lighter menstrual flow, a lighter flow is evidence that birth control creates an inhospitable environment for pre-born children — which is, of course, one of its goals. For pro-life and Christian couples — and pro-lifers and Christians in general — this is concerning information. As briefly outlined in previous chapters, there may be valid reasons for couples to avoid pregnancy, and these reasons are many and varied. While doing so, it is our responsibility to ensure that we are not endangering pre-born lives.

The sixth commandment[18] tells us: "Thou shalt

---

[18] Some denominations combine the first and second commandments, making this the 5th commandment.

not kill."[19] In forbidding murder, Christian teaching points out that this commandment requires us not only to refrain from murder but to protect the lives of our neighbours and not expose them or ourselves to any danger.[20] Jesus summarizes the second table of the law in Luke 6:31, saying: "And as ye would that men should do to you, do ye also to them likewise," and emphasizes later in this chapter that our neighbour does not only include those we love, but our enemies as well: "But I say unto you which hear, Love your enemies, do good to them which hate you, bless them that curse you, and pray for them which despitefully use you."[21] In the parable of the good Samaritan,[22] Jesus illustrates that following this commandment is required not only when it is easy to do so, but also when it may be difficult or even dangerous.

The sixth commandment is not ambiguous: we may not endanger ourselves or others. While the intent of taking birth control is most often to prevent fertilization, we cannot ignore that it can also prevent implantation. The purpose of creating birth control was to ensure that a child would not be born. While the primary purpose of birth control was to prevent ovulation, it soon became clear that

---

[19] Exodus 20:13, Deuteronomy 5:17.
[20] Heidelberg Catechism, Lord's Day 40.
[21] This point is also emphasized in the Catechism of the Catholic Church, Part 3, Article 5, 2262.
[22] Luke 10:29-37.

breakthrough ovulation[23] while on the pill can occur. The Planned Parenthood website lists effecttiveness rates of hormonal birth control between 91-99%, and that is if it is administrated properly (e.g. at the same time every day). That means pregnancy might still occur when people are taking hormonal contraceptives – the birth control fails in all three of its functions. It is safe to assume, then, that at times birth control fails to prevent ovulation, as well as to effectively prevent sperm from travelling to the fallopian tubes. When those two events happen, despite "best efforts" to prevent them, the third function of birth control, which is to create an inhospitable environment for the newly conceived child, is necessary to increase its overall effectiveness. After all, most people, physicians included, do not find it important *how* the pill works; rather, they are concerned *that* it works.

In commanding that we do not murder, the sixth commandment also commands that we do everything within our power to protect another's life.[24] Some may argue that birth control is not the only thing that may potentially harm a pre-born child. They may claim that any married woman with the potential of conceiving a child should be taking folic acid and/or a prenatal vitamin to ensure that her body is as prepared as possible to nurture a new human being. If we don't say that

---

[23] When a woman is taking a form of birth control meant to suppress ovulation and ovulation occurs, it is called "breakthrough ovulation".

[24] Heidelberg Catechism, Lord's Day 40, Question 107.

women who don't take prenatal vitamins are potentially endangering their children, why would we say that birth control endangers them? Are we not being too particular when we speak of potentially endangering children who do not even exist yet?

We should acknowledge that women have a unique responsibility since attempting to be healthy does not always affect their person only, but also the child or children they may carry within their body. However, not maintaining a healthy lifestyle or taking specific measures (e.g., folic acid, prenatal vitamins, etc.) to enrich a placenta from which the child receives his or her nutrition is *very* different from taking a drug that was created with the sole purpose of ensuring that her body is a toxic environment for a pre-born child. Hormonal birth control and the copper IUD have abortifacient capabilities, meaning that these drugs cause abortions. We cannot know exactly how many lives are ended because of these capabilities. HCG[25] (known as the pregnancy hormone) is only detectable *after* implantation—and because each form of birth control affects women differently (e.g., the IUD prevents ovulation in some women but not in others) it would be difficult, if not impossible, to assess how birth control would function in each individual case.

The Bible is clear that Christians have special responsibilities to care for the vulnerable (Proverbs 31:8-9, Isaiah 1:17, James 1:27) and that parents

---

[25] Human chorionic gonadotropin.

have special responsibilities toward their children (1 Timothy 5:8, Proverbs 13:22, Colossians 3:21, Ephesians 6:4). While a pre-born child may not exist in the moment someone takes birth control, there is still a responsibility towards a child that *may* come into existence. When a man and woman engage in intercourse, they are engaging in an act that is both unitive and procreative. Together, they become "one flesh" (Genesis 2: 24), but they also engage in an act that is procreative in its nature – the organs involved are called *reproductive* (not recreational) *organs*. It is negligent to claim that there is no responsibility towards children that may be created as a result of engaging in an act where one of the primary purposes is to conceive a child.

Some may argue that the potential for birth control to cause an abortion is minimal. After all, pregnancy does not occur every time a woman has sexual intercourse. Intercourse would have to occur on the few fertile days she has every month, with a man who has healthy sperm. If this were to happen, the birth control would have to fail to prevent ovulation *and* the cervical mucus would have to inadequately impair sperm movement and function. Isn't it extreme to refuse the use of birth control to avoid such a small risk of harm? As Randy Alcorn writes in *Does the Birth Control Pill Cause Abortions?*: "To be an abortifacient does not require that something always cause an abortion, only that it sometimes does."[26] But if sometimes is actually *rarely,*

---

[26] Alcorn, Randy. *Does the Birth Control Pill Cause Abortions?* 11th edition (2011), pg. 44.

some may feel that birth control does not carry enough of a risk to necessitate avoiding it. That is, undoubtably, the most comfortable answer to a difficult question, but is it the right one?

To what extent are parents responsible for the safety of their children? Is it extreme to avoid using birth control because it *may* cause the death of your tiny baby?

It is important to note that there is a distinct difference between taking birth control as a method of family planning or taking it as a medication. While this will be discussed in more depth in the following chapters, there are many medications, including ibuprofen (Advil), that carry some risk to a child during early pregnancy. It is important that we understand what these risks are, and when taking one or more of these medications is necessary, carefully discern when pregnancy needs to avoided. Acknowledging the risks that other medications pose to pregnancy is important, but we also need to recognize that taking a medication that was created with the purpose of addressing a medical condition is different than using a method of birth control that was created with the intent of preventing pregnancy.

Finally, we must consider the possibility that birth control can also harm an embryo *after* they have implanted in the uterine lining. If all of the mechanisms of contraception fail and the baby does implant in the uterine lining, a woman would not yet know that this has occurred and may continue using her birth control. There is little research surrounding the effects of birth control after the embryo has implanted, as conducting this type of research is ethically problematic. Most doctors insist that there is *little* risk to the child,[27] but at the same time, they do not affirm that there is *no* risk (the little risk they speak of does not include the IUD, which carries a significant risk of pregnancy complications.)[28] While most research may suggest that the risk to the baby is minimal, we need to ask the question: What is a minimal risk? Is any risk to a pre-born child unworthy of concern? In the many different situations a couple may face, this is a question that requires careful consideration.

It is important to emphasize that even if it is not our intent to end someone's life, if actions we take result in someone's death, we must face that we have a level of culpability. We know that sex can result in the conception of a child. If it is true that birth control can ensure that this child starves to death, and we continue to use it, are we following the command to prevent the hurt of our neighbour — the closest of which would be our own children — as much as possible?

---

[27] Myra Wick, M.D., "Do birth control pills cause birth defects if taken during early pregnancy?" *Mayo Clinic,* accessed October 7, 2022, https://www.mayoclinic.org/healthy-life-style/pregnancy-week-by-week/expert-answers/birth-control-pills/faq-20058376

[28] Dawn Stacey, "Taking Birth Control While Pregnant: What Happens?" *verywell health,* February 23, 2022, https://www.verywellhealth.com/will-taking-the-pill-while-pregnant-harm-the-baby-906925

4

What if pregnancy *needs* to be avoided?

"Have you ever taken the pill?" Jessica asked. "My doctor said I need to start taking it. It's either that or an IUD, and I'm uncomfortable with something staying in my body long-term."

"Why would the doctor tell you to take the pill?"

"Well, I've had two c-sections. Because of how this last pregnancy was high-risk, the doctor says I need to make sure I don't get pregnant for at least a year. A year and a half would be even better."

"Okay," Alannah said, "that makes sense. But can't you just track your cycle?"

Jessica laughed. "Yeah, that's what we were trying to do when I got pregnant. Because we don't seem to have trouble getting pregnant and tracking hasn't worked for us, the doctor says its super important that I make sure pregnancy doesn't happen too soon this time. She said the only way to be absolutely sure is if I use some kind of birth control."

***

There are legitimate reasons for couples to

avoid pregnancy. When a woman has recently had a caesarean section the doctors recommend that pregnancy be avoided for at least six months. For women who have undergone chemotherapy the recommended wait time can be anywhere from six months to five years, and in some cases, even longer. Other women have to take medications for health conditions that could be dangerous to a developing child. For many of these women, doctors recommend birth control. When a woman resists the idea, many doctors insist that birth control is the only truly effective way to avoid pregnancy, other than, of course, total abstinence. For married couples, while some situations may call for prolonged abstinence, total abstinence is not the answer, and neither is it, in most cases, a biblical one (1 Corinthians 7).

Those who argue that avoiding pregnancy within marriage is always wrong may not be seeing the whole picture. There are many couples who agree that children are a blessing from the Lord, who may have one or more children or may long to have them but must avoid getting pregnant due to health struggles. In some of these situations, getting pregnant would not only be dangerous for the mother, but it would also be dangerous for her preborn child. It is not selfish for a woman undergoing treatments to avoid pregnancy, nor is it wrong for a woman struggling with her mental health to delay pregnancy while she finds the medication she needs. Mothering children is an important task, part of which involves ensuring that a child is nurtured in a healthy environment. If a woman is not healthy, her womb may not be a safe place for a child.

Does this mean that there are some situations where a woman may use birth control? If getting pregnant while taking medications would be dangerous for a child, wouldn't it be better for a woman to take birth control and avoid getting pregnant altogether? Answering yes to this question would be the easiest way to resolve this issue if birth control did, in fact, effectively prevent pregnancy 100% of the time. However, as outlined in the previous chapters, we know that this is not the case, and we know that birth control potentially endangers the life of a child.

This leads to a difficult question: how can one effectively avoid pregnancy without using birth control? Jessica's doctor was correct in saying that the only way to effectively avoid pregnancy 100% of the time is by total abstinence. This is not necessarily the answer to every situation. However, there are times in marriage when couples must avoid having intercourse for a shorter or longer period, either for the health of the mother or the pre-born child (e.g., placenta previa). That said, there are ways to prevent pregnancy that are effective and safe for both mother and child.

The most common way to naturally avoid pregnancy would be for a woman to track her ovulatory cycle and avoid intercourse on the days when she is most fertile. This method is known as natural family planning (NFP). A woman is not able to get pregnant every day of the month. For most women, there is an approximately 7-day window where she is fertile: the five days leading up to ovulation, the day of ovulation, and the day after ovulation. It is not always easy to pinpoint exactly when ovulation occurs, as it can happen at different times for different people. For some women, tracking is as simple as downloading an app, logging the start of their menstrual cycle, and avoiding intercourse on the days the app tells them to. For others, taking ovulation tests every month is enough to tell them exactly when ovulation occurs. Many couples use these simple tracking methods and successfully avoid pregnancy.

However, some couples, as Jessica complained, track their cycles carefully and still end up pregnant. Many factors affect a woman's fertile window, and something as simple as going to bed too late one night can upset the delicate hormonal balance, causing ovulation to occur earlier or later than expected. For those who need to avoid pregnancy for health reasons, basic tracking may not be enough. However, new tracking systems developed by companies such as MIRA and Clearblue[29] are becoming more intricate and effective all the time.

An important step in using NFP effectively would be understanding how our bodies work. There are extensive programs that have been developed to help women regulate their hormones and

---

[29] Bouchard, Thomas, and Genius, Stephen, "Personal fertility monitors for contraception," *Canadian Medical Association Journal,* January 11, 2011, https://www.cmaj.ca/content/183/1/73

understand their cycles. In most cases, these programs were created to help women struggling with infertility. Because the focus is generally to pinpoint ovulation, these programs can help in the opposite way as well.

NaProTECHNOLOGY's website states that it is "a researched and published women's health science based on CrMS (cervical mucus) observations, which provides objective information on the cycle." It describes itself as "the first to network family planning with reproductive and gynecologic health monitoring and maintenance." [30] With a simple online search it is easy to find pages of testimonies from women who, through this program, learned to understand their cycles. One woman shared that: "Even though we didn't get pregnant while using the program, I recommend taking the course for anyone who needs help understanding and regulating their cycle."[31]

The Marquette method of NFP is described as "a sympto-hormonal method of natural family planning (NFP). Couples can observe signs of fertility and track that information to avoid or achieve pregnancy." This method is very effective in identifying the fertile window, using "cervical mucus observations and urinary hormone measurements," as well as "optional instructions for incorporating basal body temperature (BBT), urine luteinizing hormone (LH) tests, and urine progesterone

---

[30] "About NaProTECHNOLOGY," *NaPROTECHNOLOGY,* 2022, https://naprotechnology.com/about/
[31] * In conversation with the author.

tests to help be more precise in identifying fertility."[32] Similarly, the Billings Ovulation Method relies on cervical mucus patterns during the menstrual cycle to identify the fertile window.[33]

Many health professionals are dedicated to these methods of natural family planning. While they may involve more work by the individual than simply taking a pill at the same time every day, they are generally healthier. Understanding their hormones and how their bodies work is an important way for women to ensure that they are healthy, and an effective way to achieve or avoid pregnancy. In describing the fertility awareness-based methods of family planning, some of the advantages SHORE Centre lists are: "Allows the person with the uterus to understand their cycle and body," and "No hormones."[34] The disadvantages listed are telling: "Demands motivation, willingness," and "Requires time and effort to learn the correct use of the method."[35] What SHORE Centre does not observe is that using NFP ensures that husband and wife *share* the responsibility of avoiding pregnancy. It is good and healthy for couples to

---

[32] "The Marquette Method," *Whole Mission,* 2019-2022, https://www.mmnfp.com/marquettenfp

[33] Mayo Clinic Staff, "Cervical mucus method for natural family planning," *Mayo Clinic,* March 24, 2021, https://www.mayoclinic.org/tests-procedures/cervical-mucus-method/about/pac-20393452

[34] SHORE Centre, "Other Methods," *SHORECENTRE,* accessed October 7, 2022, https://www.shorecentre.ca/birth-control/

[35] Ibid.

work together when pregnancy must be avoided for health reasons. It is not only the woman who must be motivated and willing, but also her husband. Advocates for the Billings Ovulation Method of NFP explain that using this method can allow for "deepening unity, respect, communication, trust, and intimacy between the couple."[36]

Is NFP 100% effective? No. Is hormonal birth control 100% effective? Also no. When used correctly, birth control has very high success rates. The same goes for NFP. In fact, researchers have found that the symptothermal method of NFP "is as effective as the contraceptive pill for avoiding unplanned pregnancies if used correctly."[37] Both NFP and HBC have margins of error, and people have become pregnant while on birth control as well as when tracking their cycle. The difference between the two is that using a method of natural family planning will not intentionally or unintentionally end the life of an innocent human being, while using hormonal birth control or the copper IUD may do just that.

---

[36] Dr. Christian Vargas, "Billings Ovulation Method and deepening unity, respect, communication, trust, and intimacy between the couple," *WOOMB,* accessed October 7, 2022, https://woombinternational.org/philosophy/billings-ovulation-methodand-deepening-unity-respect-communication-trust-and-intimacy-between-the-couple/

[37] European Society for Human Reproduction and Embryology. "Natural Family Planning Method As Effective As Contraceptive Pill, New Research Finds." *ScienceDaily,* 21 February 2007, https://www.sciencedaily.com/releases/2007/02/070221065200.htm>

5

What Birth Control can do to your Body

"A stroke? But you're twenty-four!" Lydia looked at Katie in amazement. "What triggered that?"
"The doctors don't know yet. They're thinking it's some type of genetic condition."
"You definitely don't seem like someone likely to have a stroke. You're healthy, you get enough exercise. I thought this only happened to older people! Is there something you're taking that could have triggered this?"
"That's what they're trying to find out. What's been really crazy to me is that every doctor and specialist I've been to so far has assumed that I'm on birth control."
"Really? Why would they assume that?"
"Apparently, if someone my age comes in after having a stroke or with stroke-like symptoms, it's generally caused by birth control."
"Wait, birth control can cause strokes? I'm not on it, but when my doctor was trying to convince me to take it, he said any side effects would be minor. He said taking the pill was totally safe!"

***

When discouraging women from taking hormonal birth control, there is a clear moral objection based on its abortifacient capabilities. However, when explaining what the sixth commandment means, Christian teaching emphasizes that not only are we not to harm others, we are also required not to harm ourselves. Paul writes in 1 Corinthians 6:19-20: "What? know ye not that your body is the temple of the Holy Ghost which is in you, which ye have of God, and ye are not your own? For ye are bought with a price: therefore glorify God in your body, and in your spirit, which are God's." The Golden Rule[38] teaches that we ought to treat our neighbour as ourselves, which assumes that we treat ourselves with care, as Ephesians 5:29 outlines: "For no man ever yet hated his own flesh; but nourisheth and cherisheth it, even as the Lord the church." Is it reasonable to suggest that taking hormonal birth control is hurting oneself or exposing oneself to danger? There is evidence to suggest this.

What is the primary purpose of birth control? At a fundamental level, birth control is meant to disrupt the healthy functioning of the body. Psalm 139 reads: "I will praise thee; for I am fearfully and wonderfully made: Marvellous are thy works; And that my soul knoweth right well." A woman's fertility is a precious gift; from when she begins to menstruate through to menopause, her monthly cycles are evidence that her body is functioning in the way that it should. Disrupting this healthy functioning has negative side effects.

---

[38] Luke 6:31, Matthew 7:12.

The body's systems are hugely interdependent, and a woman's hormones affect her life in literally every way,[39] from energy levels and mood to who she chooses as a partner.[40] Women feel differently at different times of the month depending on the messages hormones are sending to their brain. The ovaries are a significant part of the endocrine system, and repressing ovulation upsets the natural messaging to the brain. This can lead to anything from a lower libido (sex drive) to a higher incidence of depression.[41]

Embraced by women and their doctors almost without question,[42] hormonal birth control is commonly used from ages 15 and upward,[43] with over half of women taking the pill for reasons other than preventing pregnancy.[44] Hormonal contraception and the pill in particular have been used as a band-aid solution to mitigate the symptoms of a myriad of women's health concerns from endometriosis to PCOS (polycystic ovarian syndrome). For many women, the pill successfully reduces symptoms

---

[39] IRB Media, *Summary of Sarah Hill's This is Your Brain on Birth Control,* (2022), pg. 41, published by IRB Media.

[40] Ibid., pg. 21.

[41] Ibid., 36.

[42] Ibid., 45.

[43] Guttmacher Institute, "Contraceptive Use in the United States," April 2020, https://www.guttmacher.org/fact-sheet/contraceptive-use-among-adolescents-united-states

[44] Guttmacher Institute, "Many American Women Use Birth Control for Noncontraceptive Reasons," November 15, 2011, https://www.guttmacher.org/news-release/2011/many-american-women-use-birth-control-pills-noncontraceptive-reasons.

such as painful cramping and heavy bleeding. However, it does not address the underlying causes of these conditions.

The pill, used as a bandaid solution, has resulted in a lack of information on women's health and has encouraged a somewhat lackadaisical attitude towards research in these areas.[45] Treating the healthy functioning of the body—women's fertility—as an illness that needs to be treated, and masking our body's way of telling us that something is, in fact, wrong—pain and discomfort—has consequences.

Planned Parenthood and SHORE both claim that birth control has health advantages. There is evidence that hormonal birth control can reduce the risk of ovarian cancer and endometrial cancer. However, this is exchanged for a higher incidence of breast and cervical cancer.[46] It can also help women who struggle with endometriosis—overgrowth of the uterine lining. However, for women who attempt to stop taking the pill after years of being on it, the health conditions masked by taking the pill often resurface and still need to be dealt with.

The fact that the pill can mask health conditions that ought to be dealt with immediately is one of the reasons why some people claim that the pill can

---

[45] IRB Media, *Summary of Sarah Hill's This is Your Brain on Birth Control,* (2022), pg. 46-47, published by IRB Media.
[46] National Cancer Institute, "Oral Contraceptives and Cancer Risk," February 22, 2018, https://www.cancer.gov/about-cancer/causes-prevention/risk/hormones/oral-contraceptives-fact-sheet.

cause infertility. While many studies have shown that the pill does not, in fact, cause infertility, there are several ways in which it can be instrumental in making people struggle to achieve pregnancy. The first, as mentioned, is the masking of health conditions that can be complicated and difficult to rectify. When coupled with the fact that women are often intentionally delaying pregnancy until their mid to late thirties, dealing with these conditions can take time that their biological clocks do not have.

Post-pill amenorrhea is when a woman's cycle does not return to normal for at least 6 months after she stops taking the pill or another form of hormonal contraception. Depending on how long a woman has been on birth control, it can take months or even years for a woman's cycle to be naturally regulated.[47] The pill also depletes antioxidants such as CoQ10, vitamin E, vitamin C, and selenium,[48] which are crucial to ovarian health. Finally, for women who have used the pill for longer periods of time (five years or more, which is very common, considering girls often begin taking birth control in their teens), the lining of their uterus may be thinner than for women who have

---

[47] C. Gnoth et al., "Cycle characteristics after discontinuation of oral contraceptives," *National Library of Medicine,* August 2002, https://pubmed.ncbi.nlm.nih.gov/12396560/
[48] M. Palmery et al., "Oral Contraceptives and changes in nutritional requirements," *National Library of Medicine,* July 2013, https://pubmed.ncbi.nlm.nih.gov/23852908/

not taken birth control.[49] A healthy endometrial lining is essential for implantation and sustaining the life of a baby.

Hormonal birth control upsets the natural balance of hormones in the body. While there are times when our body isn't regulating these hormones properly, these conditions need to be addressed, rather than simply masking the symptoms. The side affects of birth control are not difficult to source. Some of the "disadvantages" to hormonal birth control that SHORE Centre lists are:

- May increase risk of blood clots
- May cause irregular bleeding or spotting, breast tenderness, abdominal bloating, acne, nausea or headaches
- May cause vaginal discomfort or irritation
- Causes a decrease in bone mineral density
- Perforation of uterus may occur at insertion (rare)
- Can cause changes in menstrual bleeding pattern
- May cause emotional changes; May worsen mental health conditions[50]

Using birth control also has the potential to upset the natural balance of healthy bacteria in a

---

[49] Nayana Talukdar et al., "Effect of long-term combined oral contraceptive pill use on endometrial thickness," *National Library of Medicine,* August 2012, https://pubmed.ncbi.nlm.nih.gov/22825095/

[50] SHORE Centre, "Birth Control Options," accessed September 21, 2022, https://www.shorecentre.ca/birthcontrol/

woman's body, making her prone to candida over-growth—resulting in yeast infections which mani-fest themselves through vaginal itching and dis-comfort, burning around the vaginal opening, pain or dryness during sex, smelly discharge, and red-ness or swelling.[51] Most "resources" are quick to note, however, that there are also many risks asso-ciated with pregnancy and the post-partum period, risks which they claim exceed the risks related to birth control. The claim that there are only two op-tions, pregnancy or birth control, undermines the idea that there are ways other than birth control for women to avoid pregnancy.

Ultimately, birth control has been promoted as something that women *need*. When women believe that if they don't take birth control they *will* face an unwanted and/or unplanned pregnancy at some point in their lives, they often decide that the poten-tial health risks are worth it. Not only is this misin-formation (as outlined in Chapter 4, there *are* other ways to effectively avoid pregnancy), but it leads women to believe that nothing could possibly be worse than being pregnant.

While the health risks surrounding the use of hormonal birth control are often brushed aside, it is worth pointing out that birth control is not recom-mended to *all* women. For women who smoke and are 35 or older, stopped smoking less than a year

---

[51] Debra Sullivan R.N., "What is the link between birth con-trol and yeast infections?" *Medical News Today*, September 30, 2017, https://www.medicalnewstoday.com/arti-cles/319568#symptoms-of-a-yeast-infection

ago and are 35 or older, are very overweight, or take certain medications,[52] birth control is not advised. Further, if someone has or had blood clots in a vein (or a family history of blood clots under the age of 45), stroke or any other disease that narrows the arteries, a heart abnormality or heart disease (including high blood pressure), severe migraines, breast cancer, gallbladder or liver disease, or diabetes with complications,[53] the type of birth control, if any, that is safe to take needs to be carefully reviewed by a doctor and pharmacist. In these cases, even if pregnancy itself poses serious risks to a woman, doctors would have to recommend an alternative way to prevent pregnancy. This information suggests that there is widespread knowledge in the medical community that taking birth control can have a negative impact on a woman's health.

Interrupting the healthy functioning of our bodies is something that has serious moral implications. 1 Corinthians 3:16-17 states: "Know ye not that ye are the temple of God, and that the Spirit of God dwells in you? If any man defile the temple of God, him shall God destroy; for the temple of God is holy, which temple ye are." Hormonal birth control can cause a variety of cardiovascular issues such as stroke, deep vein thrombosis, and blood clots. It can affect mood, lead to higher incidences

---

[52] NHS, "Combined pill, Your contraception guide," July 1, 2020, https://www.nhs.uk/conditions/contraception/combined-contraceptive-pill/
[53] Ibid.

of depression, and aggravate migraine attacks.[54] These are serious health conditions that should not be overlooked.

We are called to care for our bodies. While some avoid pregnancy for legitimate reasons, many take birth control simply because it is more convenient than carefully tracking one's cycle. If hormonal birth control endangers the lives of pre-born children and can adversely affect a woman's health, isn't it necessary to look for alternative options?

---

[54] Ann Pietrangelo, "The Effects of Hormonal Birth Control on Your Body," *healthline,* January 26, 2022, https://www.healthline.com/health/birth-control-effects-on-body#migraine

6

What if birth control is needed to treat health conditions?

"What do you mean, you're taking the pill?" Marie asked. "Don't you find it makes you super moody?"
Claire sighed. "I know taking the pill isn't ideal, but I literally had no other choice."
"What do you mean?"
"Every month during my period, the bleeding was intense, and my cramps were so bad I would literally pass out when I stood up. I had to stay in bed for at least three days every month. The doctor said I had PCOS and the only way to manage it was to take birth control."
"Did it help?"
"Yes. My periods are lighter, and the cramping isn't so bad. It hasn't helped a huge amount with the acne, but that's a little better, too. I definitely struggle with mood swings still, and my energy levels aren't amazing, but at least I can function. You can't just stay in bed for three days every month."

***

In Genesis 3, the Bible outlines the fall of humanity at the instigation of the devil. In verse 16,

God pronounced the curse of the woman: "I will greatly multiply thy sorrow and thy conception; in sorrow thou shalt bring forth children ..." The difficulties surrounding a woman's menstrual cycle, the conception and carrying of children, and labour and delivery are unavoidable. However, while some pain and discomfort are expected, many underlying conditions need to be treated. The question is, how? Balancing hormones is a delicate business, and if birth control is not the answer, what is?

As mentioned in Chapter 5, there is a lack of research focused on women's health issues. Likely, this is partly due to the widespread prescription of hormonal birth control, which, rather than treating the underlying causes of these concerns, effectively masks many of their symptoms. The birth control pill *does* address many of the difficulties women face: heavy bleeding, extreme cramping, acne, irregular cycles, etc. However, the fundamental issue is not addressed, and when a woman stops taking hormonal birth control, she often finds that her symptoms resurface even more intensely than before. In recent years, more doctors — many of them female — have turned to this area of study, realizing that bandaid solutions aren't helping women understand their bodies and how to work with their cycles rather than against them.

Most of the new programs that have been introduced to deal with "women's health issues" have focused on lifestyle choices. Diet, exercise, and sleep habits play major roles in balancing a woman's hormones, something that many doctors focus on very little, if at all. One doctor, based in

Alberta, has helped patients overcome many of the symptoms of Polycystic Ovarian Syndrome (PCOS) with a focus on lifestyle changes. One woman wrote:

> I spent many years feeling hopeless about my polycystic ovarian diagnosis. Irregular and heavy periods, insulin resistance, obesity, and lack of energy were just some of the things I was experiencing... Through Dr. Genuis' expertise, she helped guide me into taking control of my health in a way that works specifically with my body. A lot of my PCOS symptoms have reversed, and I am a much healthier version of myself thanks to her guidance.[55]

Another woman had a similar story:

> When I was diagnosed with Polycystic Ovarian Syndrome, I felt hopeless. It seemed like I would never have a regular period, always be overweight, and continue down the road of insulin resistance. Through Dr. Genuis' gentle guidance and medical expertise, I was given the tools I needed to take control of my health. In making environmental and lifestyle changes, almost all of my symptoms reversed.[56]

Hormonal birth control essentially hijacks a

---

[55] Rebecca Genuis M.D., *Testimonials*, accessed September 28, 2022, https://www.rebeccagenuis.com
[56] Ibid.

woman's endocrine (hormonal) system. A naturo-pathic doctor based in Toronto explains that while birth control can produce monthly bleeds, "this approach does not address the underlying causative factors at play."[57] She explains that the causative factors are "insulin resistance, imbalanced sex hormones, overstimulation of the adrenal glands, excess inflammation or a combination of these causes."[58] This doctor also has lists of testimonials from women who have found her helpful. This does not mean these methods will work for everyone, but it does indicate that there are options other than hormonal birth control.

It is an individual responsibility to look after one's own body. Blindly and unquestioningly trusting doctors (whatever the doctor's focus) is attempting to pass this responsibility over to someone else. NaProTECHNOLOGY, previously mentioned in Chapter 4, is valuable because it can help women understand their cycle. If we don't know how our bodies are supposed to function, it can be difficult to tell if something is normal or a health concern, and further, if there are habits we can change to address negative symptoms.

There is an increasing number of books and blogs that encourage women to look for better alternatives to hormonal birth control. Some may be concerned that directing women towards healthier

---

[57] Kelly Clinning, "Polycystic Ovarian Syndrome (PCOS): Manage PCOS Symptoms Naturally," accessed September 28, 2022, https://www.kellyclinning.ca/pcos1
[58] Ibid.

and more natural methods of managing their struggles with hormones is trivializing their concerns. We are used to our health concerns being addressed during an appointment with a physician. Family doctors often play an important role in dealing with women's health issues; most doctors are deeply committed to their patients' health and well-being. However, there is an overall lack of resources provided to deal with these concerns, and many doctors have been trained to turn to birth control as the easiest way to resolve any issues. Additionally, it is important to note that the contraceptive pills market is expected to reach 20.55 billion dollars by 2026,[59] and it is safe to assume that pharmaceutical companies are not in a hurry to slash this revenue.

While we would like to believe that these companies, as well as all healthcare professionals, have our best interests at heart, it would be naive to assume that this is *always* the case—not to mention that we may have different ideas about what is, in fact, best. In taking responsibility for our health, we need to do our own research, ask our doctors clarifying questions, and read the fine print included in

---

[59] Fortune Business Insights, "Contraceptive Pills Market to reach USD 20.55 Billion by 2026; Rising Demand for Birth-control Pills from Urban Areas to Fuel Growth: Fortune Business Insights," *GlobeNewswire,* December 19, 2019, https://www.globenewswire.com/en/news-release/2019/12/19/1962675/0/en/Contraceptive-Pills-Market-to-reach-USD-20-55-Billion-by-2026-Rising-Demand-for-Birth-control-Pills-from-Urban-Areas-to-Fuel-Growth-Fortune-Business-Insights.html

the packages of our filled prescriptions. While it may be difficult for many of us to admit, we are generally more willing to pop a pill prescribed by our doctor than to change certain aspects of our lifestyle—even when we are aware that this medication comes with some negative side effects.

In saying all of the above, it is important to note that it hasn't been said that it is *always* unethical to take the pill. There are period-related health conditions that have symptoms that are incredibly severe and depressing. In cases where a woman is not sexually active, and there is no potential for an embryo to be harmed, she could take the pill to address these symptoms while seeking to address the underlying health condition. Even in these cases, though, the woman (or teenager and her parents) should be fully aware of the health risks involved.

7

Interacting with Medical Professionals

"How many children do you have?"
"This is our fourth baby."
"Four! What type of birth control have you been using?"
"We don't use birth control. I've tracked my cycle using ovulation strips between pregnancies."
"Oh boy. That explains it. In situations like yours we recommend the IUD. It's long-lasting, so you don't have to worry about taking a pill every day."
"I don't want to go on any birth control. My cycle has always been pretty consistent, so tracking has been fairly straight forward."
"There's always a chance you'll get pregnant while sexually active, and tracking is never 100% reliable. The responsible decision would be to go on birth control."

***

It is common practice, at least in Canada, for healthcare providers to ask every woman who comes in for a post-partum checkup what her birth control plan is. While for most providers this is not necessarily meant to pressure women into taking birth control when they would rather not, there are several assumptions made when this question is asked.

The practitioner is assuming that the woman is unable to track her cycle accurately enough to avoid pregnancy.

There is the assumption that the woman does not want another child—at least not for a long time.

It is inferred that the woman is willing to use whatever means necessary to ensure that pregnancy does not occur, even if it affects her own health and potentially the life and health of her baby. These are serious assumptions to make.

In a country where a woman's "choice" is championed and "reproductive freedom" is considered sacred, we must understand that our society's view of pregnancy and children is not a biblical one. Having more than two or three children is often considered irresponsible, and a fourth child may be asked if their parents "slipped up." Doctors, nurses, and random strangers do not necessarily mean to be rude or unkind: many simply do not understand the desire for—or welcoming attitude towards—more children, and often their own lifestyles would not be conducive to having a larger family. The priorities of home and family have been largely swapped for career and individualism, and children don't fit very well into the new picture.

It can be difficult to understand that those who have dedicated their lives to women and children's health may still push the use of birth control. Many of us with children have had positive experiences with doctors, nurses, midwives, and obstetrician-gynecologists: health care professionals who worked hard to ensure that we and our children came through pregnancy, childbirth, and the post-partum period safely. It can be challenging to believe that many of these same people recommend and even pressure women to go on hormonal birth control and, further, that many of these same people support abortion.

How is it possible for people to hold such opposing beliefs at the same time? When people hold beliefs or values that conflict with one another, it is called cognitive dissonance—a literal split in ideas where someone never holds these two views beside each other in order to analyze their compatibility. Dr. Fraser Fellows, who worked in London, Ontario (he retired recently), worked in labour and delivery. He also did abortions up to 23 weeks and six days and was considered a late-term abortionist. For him, and many health care providers like him, this doesn't produce the conflict of interest we may see. Heralded as a champion for woman's rights, Dr. Fellows cared for the babies women wanted and disposed of the ones they did not. He could be trusted to care for a pre-born child that was wanted because the primary concern was the mother's overall satisfaction.

Our society deems a baby worthy of care if he/she is wanted *and* convenient. A child may have been wanted, but if discovered to have a genetic abnormality, it may be considered inconvenient and, thus, disposable. A child conceived when parents were actively trying to avoid pregnancy may be considered inconvenient and, thus, disposable. A child who turns out to be a girl rather than the desired boy may be disposable. That's the way our society works. In light of this, is it really possible to blindly trust our doctors when it comes to the lives of our pre-born children?

Parents are responsible for caring for the safety of their children, both born and pre-born. Passing this responsibility off in whole or in part to medical professionals can be unsafe. While sad, it is a truth that cannot be ignored: most medical professionals do not have the same view of pre-born children that we do. We have a responsibility to protect and advocate for our children, and this means that we need to do our research *before* a doctor's visit, ask difficult questions, and encourage conversation.

When a doctor explains that a form of birth control prevents nidation, how many of us would understand that to mean the implantation of an already conceived child? When a doctor explains that birth control is only effective prior to conception, how many of us know that many in the medical community equate conception with implantation? When a doctor offers to treat a potential ectopic pregnancy with methotrexate, how many of us would know that this could potentially result in an abortion?[60] Yes, it is *easier* to trust our doctors and follow their advice, but it is potentially dangerous for our children.

---

[60] There is debate in the pro-life community about whether the use of methotrexate to end an ectopic pregnancy is ethical.

Doing our own research is crucial. As outlined in Chapter 1, we may have a different understanding of when life begins than our doctor does. Additionally, many doctors simply don't see the loss of an early pregnancy as ethically problematic and may not share this information with patients because they don't see it as significant. It is important to note that while our doctor's intent may not be to deceive, the definitions have been molded to fit a specific political agenda as early as 1976, when the American College of Obstetricians and Gynecologists changed the definition of contraceptive.[61] The fact that many pro-life people do not understand exactly how birth control works — how many people read the fine print explaining how their medications actually function? — is not something the pro-choice movement is rushing to remedy. As Randy Alcorn points out, "...a pharmaceutical company has nothing to gain by drawing attention to this information, and potentially a great deal to lose."[62] When researching for his book on the birth control pill, Alcorn discovered that "many, probably most birth control studies are not published, at least not in their entirety."[63] Why would companies marketing a product publish information that could damage their business?

Hosea 4:1-2 says: "...the LORD hath a controversy with the inhabitants of the land, because

---

[61] Alcorn, Randy. *Does the Birth Control Pill Cause Abortions?* 11th edition (2011), pg. 16.

[62] Ibid., 109.

[63] Ibid., 104.

there is no truth, nor mercy, nor knowledge of God in the land. By swearing, and lying, and killing, and stealing, and committing adultery, they break out, and blood toucheth blood." Verse 6 laments: "My people are destroyed for lack of knowledge..." In his book *The Marketing of Evil*, David Kupelian outlines how the debates surrounding marriage, family, and abortion were won by those who understood the importance of controlling the rhetoric surrounding the debate—words, their definitions, and how they are framed *matter*. When we don't understand how society views pre-born children, our ability to defend them—even our own—is crippled.

There is one final point that needs to be considered. Is it possible that we don't fully understand these issues because we don't want to? The reaction of many pro-lifers to the evidence that hormonal birth control may cause abortions has been to search for reasons why this is not true. It is *easier* to trust our medical professionals. When we wish (or need) to avoid pregnancy it is *easier* to take the prescribed birth control. It is *easier* not to research, not to ask questions, not to look for alternative solutions. But, as Christians, we are not called to do what is easy. We are called to do what is right. The Bible does not speak lightly of our responsibility to our children. 1 Timothy 5:8 reads: "But if any provide not for his own, and specially for those of his own house, he hath denied the faith, and is worse than an infidel."

8

Emergency Contraception

News Anchor: "We had some confusion on our Facebook page. A big difference between the Morning After Pill and the Abortion Pill."
"Sure! So there's definitely a big difference. The Abortion Pill that many people confuse sometimes with Plan B – it actually gets rid of a pregnancy, so it ends a pregnancy. So somebody is already pregnant when you take an Abortion Pill."
"Uh, with the Morning After Pill..."
"With the Morning After Pill, that actually prevents a pregnancy. So, if you take a Morning After Pill when you're pregnant, that's not going to make any difference. You're going to continue being pregnant. You take an Abortion Pill that will end a pregnancy."[64]

***

The above conversation played out on a news network in the United States in 2018, attempting to explain the difference between Plan B (also known as the Morning After Pill) and the Abortion Pill.

---

[64] "What is the difference between the morning after pill and the abortion pill?" *ABC10 News*, January 10, 2018, https://www.youtube.com/watch?v=3-isDIit6sk

The anchor was quick to confirm that Plan B does not end a pregnancy, but it prevents one, which is reiterated in Planned Parenthood's emergency contraception information video.[65] Plan B falls under the category of emergency contraception, which is what people take if they either forget to use a method of contraception or do not use their method of contraception correctly. It is also usually offered to someone who has been sexually assaulted, if she goes to the hospital shortly after being attacked. Emergency contraception can be taken up to five days after sex, though most forms are only really effective for three days after.

Ella, a nonhormonal pill, is considered the most effective type of emergency contraception, acting with Ulipristal Acetate, which interferes with the natural hormone progesterone. It is 85-98% effective when taken within 72-120 hours after having sex. While other forms of emergency contraception are not as effective when taken later, Ella works well up to five days after and is more effective than other forms of emergency contraception for those with a higher BMI. Ella cannot be obtained without a prescription—some healthcare workers recommend filling a prescription ahead of time to ensure it is on hand if necessary.[66] Both SHORE Centre and

---

[65] Planned Parenthood, "Emergency Contraception," accessed September 21, 2022, https://www.plannedparenthood.org/learn/morning-after-pill-emergency-contraception

[66] Nurse Liz, "Emergency Contraception (Plan B) vs Abortion Pill/What's the Difference?" May 11, 2022, https://www.youtube.com/watch?v=bHZVPWlHEXE

Rexall relay that this drug works by preventing or delaying ovulation and potentially preventing the "egg" from implanting by altering the endometrium.[67] Rexall goes on to state: "It is important to realize that once implantation has occurred and pregnancy is established, ulipristal cannot cause an abortion or harm the fetus."[68] This is emphasized in spite of the fact that later on the same page, Rexall warns that one should NOT take this medication if one "[is] or may be pregnant."[69]

There are several problems with the language used here. First, it is clearly assumed that pregnancy does not occur until *after* an embryo implants in the endometrial lining. Secondly, Rexall claims that a woman's egg is able to implant in the endometrial lining. We know that an unfertilized egg simply passes through the uterus and is expelled during a woman's period, while an egg that is fertilized with a sperm becomes an embryo. Once an embryo exists, a woman is pregnant, whether or not this new human being is able to implant in the uterine lining.

Plan B, also known as the Morning After Pill, acts with Levonorgestrel (commonly found in birth control pills), which is the synthetic version of the

---

[67] SHORE Centre, "Emergency Contraception," accessed September 27, 2022, https://www.shorecentre.ca/birthcontrol/

Rexall Pharmacy Group ULC, "Ella," accessed September 27, 2022, https://www.rexall.ca/article/drug/view/id/7210/

[68] Ibid.

[69] Ibid.

hormone progesterone. It is 88-95% effective when taken within 72 hours (three days) after intercourse but can be taken up to five days after, though with reduced effectiveness. It is an over-the-counter drug that generally costs around thirty dollars. The Planned Parenthood information video states that it "mainly works by stopping sperm from meeting with an egg."[70] However, the Plan B website lists the following three functions:

When taken correctly... Plan B works by:
- Temporarily stopping the release of an egg from the ovary (ovulation).
- Preventing fertilization.
- Preventing a fertilized egg from attaching to the uterus by changing the uterine lining.[71]

Directly after listing this information, the website firmly states, "Plan B is not an abortion pill—if you take Plan B, you will not be terminating a pregnancy."[72] Once again, note the term "fertilized egg" and the emphasis on pregnancy beginning at the point of implantation rather than fertilization.

Other brands of over-the-counter pills include: Next choice, My Way, Take Action, Option 2, Preventeza, My Choice, Aftera, CONTINGENCY

---

[70] Planned Parenthood, "Emergency Contraception," accessed September 21, 2022, https://www.plannedparenthood.org/learn/morning-after-pill-emergency-contraception

[71] Plan B, "How does Plan B prevent pregnancy?" accessed September 21, 2022, https://planb.ca/en/how-plan-b-works/

[72] Ibid.

ONE, and EContra. These are all most effective when used within three days of having vaginal sex. SHORE Centre explains that most of these pills cost between $21 and $45, and "all work similarly to the birth control pill by preventing ovulation, thickening cervical fluid and thinning the lining of the uterus."[73] The fine print included in the package selling CONTINGENCY ONE reiterates these functions:

- CONTINGENCY ONE acts as an emergency contraceptive by preventing the release an egg from the ovary, or preventing sperm and egg from uniting. In addition,
- CONTINGENCY ONE may prevent the fertilized egg from attaching to the wall of the uterus. CONTINGENCY ONE is not effective once a pregnancy has started, that is once the fertilized egg has attached to the wall of the uterus.
- CONTINGENCY ONE does not cause an abortion.[74]

Like Plan B, these pills contain the medicinal ingredient Levonorgestrel.

The close relationship between hormonal birth control and emergency contraception is clear, as a combination of oral contraceptives can also be used

---

[73] SHORE Centre, "Emergency Contraception," accessed September 27, 2022, https://www.shorecentre.ca/birthcontrol/

[74] Mylan Pharmaceuticals ULC, "Part III: Consumer Information CONTINGENCY ONE," *Manufacturer's Standard,* March 9, 2018.

as emergency contraception. While it is recommended only with the oversight of a doctor, a higher dose of the birth control pill can be taken to act as emergency birth control, a method known as Combo OCP.[75] This method is not as popular as it contains estrogen as well as progestin, which can cause nausea, vomiting, headaches, and other side effects.

The Copper IUD is listed as one of the most effective methods of emergency contraception. Still, its effectiveness is hampered by the necessity of having to book a doctor's appointment within a few days of having intercourse. Getting in to see a doctor on short notice is difficult, and an IUD cannot be inserted by oneself. When inserted within five days of intercourse, the Copper IUD is 99.5% effective. The Copper IUD creates a toxic environment for sperm and also prevents any "fertilized eggs" from attaching to the uterine wall.[76]

Some Christians and pro-lifers may wonder why this chapter was included in a book focused on the way hormonal birth control potentially prevents pregnancy. While birth control is a more controversial topic in many churches, emergency contraception is known to potentially cause abortion. This is interesting because of the similarity of both

---

[75] Healthwise Staff, "Emergency Contraception," *MyHealthAlberta Network*, June 16, 2021, https://myhealth.alberta.ca/Health/Pages/conditions.aspx?hwid=tb1838

[76] Brampton Womens Clinic, "What is an IUD? Choosing which one is best for you," October 29, 2021, https://www.bramptonwomensclinic.com/what-is-an-iud-choosing-which-one-is-best-for-you/

contents and function between birth control and emergency contraception: they use similar—or identical—drugs that function in the same three ways. Preventing implantation seems to be a more obvious goal of emergency contraception. Yet, in reading the information published by those who create and/or supply these drugs, in most cases, it is emphasized that the primary function is to prevent fertilization. As with birth control, preventing implantation is mentioned as something the drug *may* do, but not as its primary function. This is significant. While studies show that the endometrial lining is significantly affected by the synthetic hormones contained in both hormonal birth control and emergency contraception, [77] companies attempt to brush this off as simply a *potential* function. Yet, doctors will readily acknowledge that within the fertility world the endometrial lining plays a *key role* in encouraging a healthy pregnancy. While the optimal thickness of the endometrial lining for a woman undergoing an IVF cycle was found to be around 10mm,[78] the average thickness of the lining for women on oral contraceptives was

---

[77] Nayana Talukdar et al., "Effect of long-term combined oral contraceptive pill use on endometrial thickness," *National Library of Medicine,* August 2012, https://pubmed.ncbi.nlm.nih.gov/22825095/

[78] Ioannis Gallos et. al. "Optimal endometrial thickness to maximize live births and minimize pregnancy losses: Analysis of 25, 767 fresh embryo transfers," *National Library of Medicine,* October 6, 2018, https://pubmed.ncbi.nlm.nih.gov/30366837/

4mm.[79]

When the TV anchors claimed that there was a difference between the Morning After Pill and the Abortion Pill, they were correct. In Canada, the abortion pill is sold under the name Mifegymiso, a two-step drug regimen. The first drug, containing Mifepristone — also known as RU-486 — blocks the production of progesterone, which breaks down the endometrial lining, essentially starving the implanted embryo of nutrients. The second drug contains Misoprostol — also called Zitotec 200 — which, with Mifepristone, causes severe cramping and contractions, often accompanied by heavy bleeding, which expels the baby from the uterus.[80]

The anchors stated that this pill could be controversial because it can end a life that has *already begun*, which, they claim, is what makes it different from the Morning After Pill. All of this depends on when life begins, as outlined in Chapter 1. Science tells us that life begins at fertilization, which means that while the Abortion Pill effectively ends the life of a more developed child, the Morning After Pill and other methods of emergency contraception can end the life of that same child, just at an earlier stage of development.

---

[79] Jason Abbott, "Oral contraceptives maintain a very thin endometrium before operative hysteroscopy," *JMIG,* September 1, 2006, https://www.jmig.org/article/S1553-4650(06)00232-9/fulltext#relatedArticles
[80] Planned Parenthood, "The Abortion Pill," *plannedparethood.org,* accessed September 27, 2022, https://www.plannedparenthood.org/learn/abortion/the-abortion-pill.

9

The Culture War

The debate surrounding contraception and birth control has always been heated and would be so even if hormonal birth control did not have abortifacient capabilities. Christians have long debated the meaning of sex, specifically, sex within marriage. The idea that sex is both unitive *and* procreative made many thinkers uncomfortable with intentionally removing one of these purposes—the conception of children—from the equation. This debate is still ongoing. As Christians, understanding the role birth control has played in causing our culture to deviate from the values we are called to cherish and defend is critical. Why has our culture embraced birth control so wholeheartedly? Why is any debate around this topic seen as a direct attack on women's rights? Why is the Western world so devoted to the idea of universally available birth control that they pour billions of dollars into making it available all around the world? These aren't easy questions to ask or answer, but they are important ones.

Before abortion became the sacred right of feminists fighting for "women's rights," the fight to decriminalize the use of contraception was center-stage. Margaret Sanger, the founder of Planned Parenthood, is credited with coining the term birth control. As a nurse, Sanger watched women struggle with pregnancy, childbirth, and large families and stated that she also treated women who were damaged by illegal abortions. Sanger felt that "female control of contraception was nothing less than a precondition to the emancipation of women. Since women disproportionately bore the burden of pregnancy and child-rearing, she believed women should have a contraceptive they alone controlled."[81]

The problems Sanger came into contact with were legitimate, even if we disagree with her solution. The idea that women need to be in sole control of their fertility is a damaging one. Men and women were created to complement each other; one cannot conceive a child without the other. Attempting to remove the man from the equation has, in many cases, simply allowed him to absolve himself of any responsibility when the woman he has had sex with becomes pregnant. After all, *she* is in control, so the fact that she is pregnant is now *her* problem. Helping women who struggled with large families and complicated pregnancies should have involved encouraging more communication between couples rather than less.

---

[81] PBS, "The Pill and the Women's Liberation Movement," *pbs.org,* accessed October 7, 2022, https://www.pbs.org/wgbh/americanexperience/features/pill-and-womens-liberation-movement/

Sanger's goal in championing contraception was not just to "liberate women." She had a deep concern regarding population growth, and had a decided dislike for certain populations. While Planned Parenthood defended its founder for years, its president and chief executive, Alexis McGill Johnson, wrote a piece for The New York Times in 2021, titled, "I'm the Head of Planned Parenthood. We're Done Making Excuses for Our Founder."[82] While refusing to say that Sanger was actually a racist, Johnson admits to the following significant actions:

> Sanger spoke to the women's auxiliary of the Ku Klux Klan at a rally in New Jersey to generate support for birth control. And even though she eventually distanced herself from the eugenics movement because of its hard turn to explicit racism, she endorsed the Supreme Court's 1927 decision in Buck v. Bell, which allowed states to sterilize people deemed "unfit" without their consent and sometimes without their knowledge — a ruling that led to the sterilization of tens of thousands of people in the 20th century.[83]

Due to these views of the woman who is known as

---

[82] Alexis McGill Johnson, "I'm the Head of Planned Parenthood. We're Done Making Excuses for Our Founder," *New York Times,* April 17, 2021, https://www.ny-times.com/2021/04/17/opinion/planned-parenthood-mar-garet-sanger.html

[83] Ibid.

one of the "mothers" of the birth control pill (the other being Katharine McCormick, a woman Sanger convinced to fund the development of the pill by medical researcher Gregory Pincus), [84] it should not be surprising that Sanger backed human trials of the birth control pill in Puerto Rico, "where as many as 1,500 women were not told that the drug was experimental or that they might experience dangerous side effects."[85] Sanger was also associated with Lothrop Stoddard, a member of the Ku Klux Klan who wrote a white supremacist book titled *The Rising Tide of Color*. Sanger appointed Stoddard to the board of the Birth Control League, the parent organization of Planned Parenthood. In her book *The Pivot of Civilization*, Sanger "advocated for the elimination of 'human weeds' and called for 'the cessation of charity, for the segregation of morons, misfits, and maladjusted,' in addition to the sterilization of 'genetically inferior races.'"[86]

---

[84] PBS, "The Pill and the Women's Liberation Movement," *pbs.org*, accessed October 7, 2022, https://www.pbs.org/wgbh/americanexperience/features/pill-and-womens-liberation-movement/

[85] Alexis McGill Johnson, "I'm the Head of Planned Parenthood. We're Done Making Excuses for Our Founder," *New York Times*, April 17, 2021, https://www.nytimes.com/2021/04/17/opinion/planned-parenthood-margaret-sanger.html

[86] Quoted in Jonathon Van Maren's article, "Despite public distancing, Planned Parenthood still continues Margaret Sanger's work—killing children at a profit," *LifeSite News*,

The ideas Sanger espoused were shocking, and yet she was vehemently defended for decades. Her dedication to freeing women through the availability of birth control made her almost untouchable — our society is so committed to protecting our so-called right to control our own bodies that we are willing to gloss over these glaring shortcomings. Is it surprising, then, that there is also a large effort to conceal the abortifacient effects of birth control?

The concerns Sanger had that a growing population would soon overwhelm the globe, resulting in mass natural disasters and an alarming lack of resources, are concerns that still fuel the idea that birth control is both good and necessary. Population control is one of the primary reasons birth control has been a focus of humanitarian aid by the Western world. In her book *Target Africa,* Obianuju Ekeocha outlines how birth control has been pushed on the African people. She explains that Western leaders have effectively "instill[ed] fear in African leaders by painting a vivid picture of their countries at the sharp edge of environmental destruction, natural resource depletion, hunger, poverty, pandemic, and disorder."[87]

While many Western countries fall well below the population replacement rate of 2.1 children per

---

April 20, 2021, https://www.lifesitenews.com/blogs/despite-public-distancing-planned-parenthood-still-continues-margaret-sangers-work-killing-children-at-a-profit/?utm_source=editor_picks&utm_campaign=standard
[87] Obianuju Ekeocha, *Target Africa: Ideological Neocolonialism in the Twenty-First Century,* Ignatius Press, San Fransisco, 2018, pg. 32.

couple, most African countries are well above this.[88] This means that Western solutions to the alleged population crisis would need to "rely heavily on a single-minded strategy that entails removing or drastically reducing the source of population growth in Africa—female fertility."[89] When high-profile couples such as Prince Harry and Meghan Markle are given awards for their "environmentally friendly" decision to limit their family to two children,[90] it's not surprising that population alarmists would pay special attention to the growing population in Africa.

There are several concerns regarding the focus on contraception in aid plans to Africa. The first is that it is not likely that African women will be fully informed about the implications of taking birth control. Ekeocha writes:

> They will not be told about failure rates, adverse side effects, and the increased risks of cancer and heart disease. They will not be told that

---

[88] Mariam Saleh, "African countries with the highest fertility rate in 2020," *statista,* April 14, 2022, https://www.statista.com/statistics/1236677/fertility-rate-in-africa-by-country/

[89] Obianuju Ekeocha, *Target Africa: Ideological Neocolonialism in the Twenty-First Century,* Ignatius Press, San Fransisco, 2018, pg. 32.

[90] Maria Noyen, "Meghan Markle and Prince Harry win $695 award from environmental charity for limiting family to 2 children," *Insider,* July 12, 2021, https://www.insider.com/meghan-markle-prince-harry-environmental-award-two-kids-2021-7

promiscuity itself is the leading cause of sexually transmitted diseases, which hormonal contraceptives such as the pill and patch do nothing to prevent. Given that women in Western societies are left in the dark about these things, the chances that African women will be respected enough to be given the facts are rather slim.[91]

The primary focus of aid should be on slashing maternal mortality rates through improved health care, providing information on natural family planning methods, and campaigning against degrading and dangerous practices such as child marriage and female genital mutilation. Instead, women are given birth control with little or no information on how it works and how it will affect them in areas where the healthcare systems are not equipped to deal with any negative side effects.[92]

Another concern with this so-called aid is the imposition of the idea that contraception will break the cycle of poverty, both without proof and without consultation with the people we are attempting to aid. Ekeocha writes: "But in their single-minded obsession to reduce the fertility rate of women in sub-Saharan Africa, the one important consideration the experts have omitted is the desired fertility

---

[91] Obianuju Ekeocha, *Target Africa: Ideological Neocolonialism in the Twenty-First Century,* Ignatius Press, San Fransisco, 2018, pg. 42.
[92] Ibid., 57.

rate of the women in question."[93] In refusing to acknowledge that the value systems of many of the cultures in Africa center on life and children as a beautiful gift, the Western world imposes its values on communities that do not want them. This, Ekeocha points out, is cultural colonialism, decisively stating: "The insistence on reducing the population of Africa, no matter what the cost to the Africans themselves, is racism, imperialism, and colonialism disguised as philanthropy."[94]

In light of all of this information, we again ask: Why? Why is our society so committed to the use of birth control? Birth control has allowed for a divorce between sex and pregnancy, has encouraged sexual promiscuity, and, in so doing, has played a part in the current explosion of sexually transmitted diseases.[95] It has negatively affected women's health and endangers the lives of their children. To summarize, it has played an instrumental role in the systematic breakdown of the natural family that has played out over the last decades. The brokenness we see all around us is the result of sin, and Satan is actively working to destroy anything that remains of the beauty given to us in Paradise. Hormonal birth control has aided this mission, and we

---

[93] Ibid., 37.
[94] Ibid., 57.
[95] Pam Belluck, "Contraceptive Used in Africa May Double Risk of H.I.V." *The New York Times,* October 3, 2011, http://www.ny-times.com/2011/10/04/health/04hiv.html?_r=1&page-wanted=all

are all suffering as a result. As Jesus warns in Matthew 24:12: "And because iniquity shall abound, the love of many shall wax cold." Love between men and women, and parents and their children, has been replaced by the so-called "free love" of the sexual revolution. But there is no such thing as free love. Someone must pay, and the first to suffer are always the most vulnerable—the children.

Conclusion

Conversations surrounding family planning are often complicated—because life is complicated. Every situation is unique, and while couples can seek outside advice, ultimately, their specific situation requires them to make personal decisions. There aren't easy answers to the question of when we are permitted to avoid pregnancy, but there are clear directives for how we may *not* go about doing so. We may never endanger the lives of ourselves or others. While some may easily accept the idea that pro-lifers should generally avoid the use of hormonal birth control, others may struggle, particularly those with more urgent reasons to avoid pregnancy. We cannot take these concerns lightly. Our lives are precious, and we have a responsibility to care for our physical and mental health. But we are not permitted to attempt to erase the role of Providence in our lives. As Randy Alcorn wrote:

> We have to weigh the increased 'risk' of having a child, a person God calls a blessing, against the possibility of killing a child, an act God calls an abomination. No matter where a Christian stands on the birth control issue, we should surely be able to agree that the possibility of having a child is always better than the possibility

of killing a child.[96]

Even more important than communication between spouses when it comes to family planning is the desire to follow the directive in 1 Corinthians 10:31, "Whether therefore ye eat, or drink, or whatsoever ye do, do all to the glory of God." These decisions cannot be made without prayer, asking God for wisdom and direction. Nothing is outside of God's control, and as we read time and again throughout Scripture, He is a God Who answers prayer. Our daily struggles with health and family can and must be laid at His feet, and there is forgiveness with Him if we have made decisions in the past that we now regret. May the lives of our children, born and pre-born, be precious to us, as they are in the eyes of God. As Alcorn emphasized in his book, God's Word ought to be the last one:

> I call heaven and earth to record this day against you, that I have set before you life and death, blessing and cursing: therefore choose life, that both thou and thy children may live (Deuteronomy 30:19).[97]

---

[96] Alcorn, Randy. *Does the Birth Control Pill Cause Abortions?* 11th edition (2011), pg. 156.
[97] Ibid., 166.